1

Contents

Introduction   6

About Me   7

Know Yourself   8

Let's Begin   11

Discovering You   60

Belief Busting   80

Trigger Driver Behaviour   87

Ownership   96

Yes   101

Energy   107

What Will You Do NOW?   116

Feedback   129

Choices   135

References & Extras   137

50 Ways to Change

2019

Whatever you think, you are not wrong!

50 Ways

to

Change

By Wendy Smith

Introduction

This book is dedicated to all of you who want to create change in your life. For years I have studied with many different teachers, read their philosophies and followed their guidance which has led me to this point of creating a 50 step guide to personal development. Experience has shown me that there is nothing like experience. Through mistakes, failures and successes I have found that following some simple guidelines and knowledge can lead to a happier fulfilled life and the realisation of the potential we all hold within us. This is my personal collection of favourite self help tips that are to the point with no fuss. The quick fix guide to pioneering personal change.

Dedicated to my wonderful teachers and mentors, friends and family plus all the curious people I have interacted with on my travels so far.

Kathryn Temple, John Phillips, Karen Szabo, Penny Warn, Bob Bhania, John & Kathleen LaValle, Richard Bandler, Mick Stott, my sister Helen and my Mum & Dad - the wisdom of you all I carry today guiding me to make better choices and challenging my knowledge to help me grow.

About Me

I became interested in personal development following a road traffic accident in 1989. The prognosis was that I would never walk again after suffering a spinal injury and spinal cord lesion. I spent 8 months in hospital and walked out on crutches. My life then became a tangled mess of frustration anger and low self esteem, lost and unsure what the future held I knew I had 2 choices. So I took the hard one, get better. This led me on a 30 year journey (which is still going) to creating change within my life. I studied NLP, Neurology, EFT and Psychology, I became a Paralympic wheelchair basketball player, passed my level 3 coaching award and then proceeded to become a basketball tutor. Through frustration and the innate ability to quit when I have had enough I ended up becoming self employed and developing the businesses that I have now finding self worth and value which has led me to feeling balance within my body and mind again. Admittedly, I am still on walking sticks yet hold the attitude that I will run again.. or die trying.

My life is full of good friends and great family. Work is enjoyable and filled with value. What more could you ask for?

Know Yourself

How many personal development books have you read? 5, 10, 15 or more. Have you found it takes you forever to reach the point and understand the learning? If you have, then this book is perfect for you. This is my personal collection of tips and knowledge that I have acquired and contemplated over the past 30 years.

So how did this come about? It was November 2017 and I was sat in Starbucks inside the Renaissance hotel Las Vegas, waiting for my colleague so we could go into the 'Go Pro' conference. As I sat there waiting, sipping my coffee I had the thought "how can I help others today"? and that was it, I got out my notebook and wrote this book.

It occurred to me at that point how I had spent hours and hours reading books that seemed to leave the key point until the last page. The majority of these books also appeared to leave out what I now consider some important factors to create transformational change on the inside and also how to apply them.

You are not what you currently think you are... well, actually you are (thoughts create things), what I mean is that you are a collection of powerful atoms with more bang than a nuclear bomb and these atoms form the community of 'you'. Just imagine that for a moment, the power you have in your cells!

"Question it all and become curious. Everything you know is currently what you have been told… do you believe it?"

How are you using that power? Do you ever think about the tiny particles we are made of and how they form this amazing system that we walk about in? You have 3 super computers on board of this system, heart, stomach and brain, these regulate and support you in life. The system you walk about in is designed to support your every thought. What are you thinking yourself into? Your thoughts are powerful energy signals that transmit information to the system and beyond. Be conscious of what you think because it comes back to you quickly. You are a walking 4DX movie theatre creating your own experience and projecting it out into the world, are you using it to create the experience you want? Or are you blindly following your autopilot pre programmed responses, not living the life you want to live.

Every moment of everyday you have multitudes of choices available to you, are you aware of the choices you are making or are you just reacting to situations and emotional responses? Do you ever sit and listen to your intuition and allow it guide you through the process of decision making? This onboard guidance system is like gold dust, the more you use it the stronger it becomes and you may even find that your life begins to flow.

Stop sleep walking and wake up to the potential you hold within you now!

Let's Begin

1. You have 5 senses, according to modern day science we have a minimum of 21 but lets stick with the 5 for now.   Sight, sound, touch, taste, smell.   The reason they are called senses is because it is how we make sense of our environment. You may think that this is common knowledge, yet most people have never considered what this means at a deeper level. Think about it, our universe is made up of energy, everything comes from the same energy... so how do we know what we should be seeing, hearing, tasting, touching and smelling? Through our senses, a combination of filters with specific functions make sense of this information as it comes in.   These vary within individuals and some can become extremely sensitive for some people.   If you think about yourself now, which senses are you most aware of?   Tune into the body and just notice what you notice, is it sound or feeling, sight or smell?

2. You are a supercomputer processing information at a staggering amount per second. The current estimation is that you filter 40 million+ bits of information per second down to 2000 of usable content for your mind to work with. This brings up the question.. what are you missing?   Without wandering into the realm of philosophy, this

always makes me curious as to who is at the programming end of what we make sense of? What I mean is, who decides what objects look like so we can make sense of them? But this is not a philosophy book so I will just leave you mulling that one over?

"You are the biggest super computer on the planet, are you making good use of yourself?"

"You see in black and white, upside down, in 2D…. what do you really know about the world?"

3. People see in black and white, 2 dimension and upside down. Are you looking at upside down images now that are black and white and flat? Curious thought isn't it? This brings me back to the thought of what actually are we seeing and how do we know what it is, the brain is a fascinating bit of kit that is amazing at filling in blanks and deciphering code… begin to be curious.

"All day long you are sieving and sorting, what is your main focus?"

4. Your mind is a filter. Every second of every day your mind is filtering information rapidly. The filters of the mind come in many different shapes and forms, some simple examples would be; memories, experiences, values, beliefs, time, space, identity, preferences, personality aspects (introvert, extrovert, pain driven, pleasure driven, same, difference), these all play a part in what

your mind decides to use as relevant to you in your daily life. Think of these like a map that helps you navigate day to day life without having to analyse every single thing in your experience. Can you imagine how much time you would waste if you had to decipher everything at all times throughout the day, you would never get anything done let alone get out of the house. You are an autopilot system that runs with a programmed sat nav.

"What are your autopilot responses, what do you do that you don't know you are doing?"

"You get what you think about… be conscious of what you are thinking"

5. The mind is a deletion, distortion and generalisation expert, happily removing anything from your environment that is of no relevance in that present moment and focusing in on the things that are really important to you in life. The good, the bad and the ugly.

"Energy flows where the focus goes"

6. Deletion happens to avoid total system overload, think about driving a car or walking to work, you cannot remember everything that was on the route you will only ever remember a specific amount of detail. Are you aware of the temperature of your left foot? Only when I ask you, unless your feet are freezing or burning :) There are so many things in your space that you are not focused on because they are of no

meaning at the moment, take a minute to look around you and notice what you have not been noticing. Look at the floor, the walls, the people, the sky, allow yourself to become curious and interested in the things that your mind is purposefully deleting, this will expand the mind and open up your perspective. It will also help you realise how powerful the brain is.

Are you distorting your current experience?

7. Distortions can be beneficial yet they can also be extremely unhelpful. They are those moments when something is mistaken for something it is not. A personal prejudice that alters our perception. Think of arachnophobia, to some people spiders are just spiders doing a good job, to those with a phobia of spiders they can appear huge and terrifying. We also can hear people speak linguistic distortions i.e. "this relationship isn't working", the speaker has taken a process (relating) and turned it into a thing (relationship), to pull apart the distortion you would ask "tell me how we are not relating?" They have distorted the whole process, when there is maybe a couple of aspects that are not satisfactory. We also distort what we hear, how many times have you

misheard words or a complete sentence that someone has said to you?

Is everything always going wrong, all the time, with everyone? …. Really?

8. Think of generalisations like judgements that we perceive to be true. Easy starters are things like doors and windows, we all know you push a door to open it right? How many of you have pushed a pull door? The same with windows, we generalise that they will all open the same. Linguistic generalisations would be things like "no one cares about my work", "everybody always puts me down". The best way to break a linguistic generalisation is to challenge it, "everybody?" "no one cares?" is that really true, where is the evidence? People who generalise lots also tend to delete many positive aspects from their map, challenging someone can really help them see and experience more in their world than what they are perceiving. We have all heard people say "everything always goes wrong". What are your generalisations? Are they helping or hindering you? Challenge them now.

"Awareness is the key to change, start becoming aware"

9. You are the best music player on the planet! A programmable iPod for the entertainment of others. Did you know that between the age of 0-7 years old you are in a brainwave state of theta? What this means is that you are basically trotting around in a state of hypnosis, soaking up experience around you and mimicking those whom you are watching. This is powerful information, you spend the first 7 years of your life being programmed by other people, everybody else is putting music on your iPod teaching you how to do life and you have little to no choice of what goes on your play list. What are you listening to? Does the music sound good? Be very aware of this process because when you reach about 7 years old, you press play and start dancing. How many people do you hear utter the words "I can never change, it's just how I am?" Think for a moment about all the things you do and think, are they yours?

"If it is not working, change it"

10. What are you dancing to? Is it a funky little number that feels good or does it sound horrendous and you find you are having trouble dancing? It is worth reviewing this track list and deciding what you want to keep and what you would like to delete, you are the product of others until you become aware of this and sometimes people can go through the whole of their life never really exploring the true potential of self. Until you discover what you want/believe in life, your life is an autopilot program created by other people running 90% of what you do. Scary thought! Make a list and start working out what is supporting you and what is limiting you. What do you say or do that sounds or looks like those around you? Question it and start to become the you that you really want to be.

"Your'e not what you do, you are what you believe"

11. People are not what they do, they are what they believe. What an odd statement you might say, well, just think about it for a moment, if someone believed they could create success what do you think their behaviour would be like on a daily basis? Would they lay in bed hitting the snooze button for hours? Would they have negative self talk? Would they walk around with a frown blaming circumstances for their life choices? There is a big fat 'lie' in the middle of belief and it is worth checking out the 'lies' that you are telling yourself on a daily basis. Remember that all your beliefs are stored on your iPod, challenge them, change them, evaluate them to see if they fit with where you want to go in life. Becoming aware of our stored belief systems allows us to own and change them, we do not have to live by past limitations, you have the choice to choose a new way of doing things.

"Choice is free, give yourself a gift and make a different choice"

12. Every second of every day you have a choice to think, do, feel, say something different. People sometimes think that they have no choice, you hear it all the time. Is that really true though? You have a choice to eat the burger or not, drink the drink or not, say the words or not, feel the anxiety/excitement or not, how many times a day do you say that you have no choice? What a powerless place to be all day in the land of no choices, what would happen if you decided now to give yourself 3 choices for every action you are about to take? When someone questions you or asks you to do something, the food you are about to eat, the conversation you are having in your head, if you could stop and give yourself 3 options, what would change with the outcome? For 7 days I challenge you to stop yourself in your tracks and make different choices, give yourself options and do something different. Maybe walk a different way to work or not listen to the news first thing, get up instead of snoozing, say no to someone instead of yes, try it and see for yourself how many options you have in life.

Are your crew on board with the Captain?

13. You are a massive cruise liner sailing the ocean. On board there is a captain and a crew. Think of the captain for the sake of this book we will call the conscious thought process (you will learn about the power of your thoughts throughout the book), this part deals with about 2000 bits of usable information a second and gives orders to the crew (unconscious), the crew deals with about 40,000,000+ bits of information a second (according to current science). The captain gives an order and the crew has to follow, what orders are you giving the crew all day? You will hear me say a lot "be conscious of what you are thinking because you get what you think about", we have thousands of thoughts a day that just drift through without being checked (autopilot), when you hear one that is unhelpful just give it a moment to decide whether that is something you want in your future, if not change it. Now many people say let the thoughts come and go like clouds and to a certain extent I agree, however, if there is a persistent thought that is causing a negative result in life I would suggest spending an amount of time changing the thought to a more supportive one, if you do this consistently the thought will

create a new pathway and the old one will dissipate. It can be a challenge, but totally worth the effort.

"Inside of everyone there is a set of actions taking place at an unconscious level"

14. People are not what they do, they are the result of what is running on the inside. All behaviours are driven by belief/emotion and as you know already our beliefs are (well the majority) installed at an early age. It is true also that we develop other beliefs as we go through life. Experiences can change beliefs really quickly and so can intense emotional states. Sometimes we just decide to challenge a belief and make a conscious shift. Have you ever had a moment where you just decided to do something that you previously thought you couldn't and then discovered you could? What did that feel like? If you cannot remember a time, then go out now and create one, experiment with possibilities and notice what you can achieve.. I mean, the word impossible is just stating 'I am possible'. Enjoy the exploration, you are only limited by your own thinking.

What is important to you?

15. Discovering your values is a powerful exercise and can guide you through life in a way that allows you to feel satisfied at all times. To find out what your values are ask yourself this question in all aspects of your life. "What is important to me about ......?". These should be one word answers and are your guide to fulfilment. Examples would be; Work - trust, honesty, loyalty, fun. Relationships - honesty, fun, sharing. Friends - trust, honesty, laughter. When you have a good list of your values then ask yourself why these aspects are important to you. The 'why' will give you your motivation for life. Once you know your own values in life ask your friends and associates, you will quickly discover that everybody has a different motivation in life and their values differ greatly. Understanding this can end conflict and help develop deeper relationships with all the people you interact with. Do you know your partners relationship values? Do you know your colleagues values? Do you know your friends values? If you want deeper connections in life then find out what makes people tick.

What would be different in your life if you stopped judging others?

16. No blame and no judgement. Everyone is doing the best they can with what they have on their iPods. How often do you judge people? The common saying is "I would never do that, why are they doing that?" How many times do you hear people judge others based on their own perspective. This is a subject that when you really get the hang of can make your life so much easier. Do you judge people by what they wear, where they work, how they speak, colour of their skin, the car they drive, where they live? We all do it and when we recognise this we can do something about it. First of all, write a list of all of the judgements you hold that you currently know about. Be honest with yourself too. Now write down where these judgements came from, did they come from your parents, school, teachers, siblings, friends, tv? Then ask yourself these questions based around all of your judgements. "Will I be happier if I drop these?" "How have they served me in the past?" "Have I missed opportunities by judging others?" "If I knew I was being judged all day every day, how would I feel?" "What is the positive purpose of judgement?" "What is the negative outcome of judgement?"

"What would be different about my day if I did not judge others?"   Now spend 7 days listening to yourself when you judge others and make the decision (if you want to) to stop and give an opportunity to yourself and someone else.

"Sight, Sound, Touch, Smell, Taste"

17. Unless you have lived in a hole somewhere your whole life you will know that people learn in different ways. Visually, auditory, kinaesthetically and ad (audio digitally). Some people have a preference for watching to learn, some people have a preference for listening, some people have a preference for doing and some people have to have lists and processes to follow. Which one do you prefer?   We tend to have 2 main preferences and the others are lesser, although some people operate utilising all 4 in unison. Spend some time working out how you take in information best, does a powerpoint give you a headache? Does too much chatter get on your nerves? Are you distracted by the movement of others or do you need to move? Have you ever noticed those people who are constantly twiddling a pen or tapping their foot, kinaesthetic?   Are there any people in your family or who you work

with that doodle all the time? Become more aware of those around you and how they learn, this will help you help others get a better result and lead to developing better relationships too.

*"A wise man once said…
your ears never get you in
trouble. Listen and learn"*

18. Did you also know that people tend to speak in a similar way to how they learn? Have you ever had a conversation with someone and found it difficult to build rapport or grasp the concept of what they are talking about? This could be something as simple as not understanding the words they are using due to them talking in a different system to you. Visual people would use phrases like "I can see it from your point of view", audio speakers would say "I hear what you are saying", kinaesthetic people would use "I get where you are coming from", ad (audio digital) would utilise "I understand the process". Take some time to listen to your friends, family and colleagues and see if you can become aware of the systems they talk in. Some people will naturally use multiple systems, when you become flexible with your language and use the same as

the people you are communicating with then you will find building deeper relationships a pleasure.

Do you listen or are you just waiting to talk?

19. The skill of listening is definitely a skill. How often do you half listen to other people when they are talking and end up saying "sorry can you repeat that?" The majority of people are just queuing up what they are going to say rather than actively listening to the person they are talking to or they are drifting off in their mind thinking about other stuff. How many times have you felt undervalued because the person you are talking to is on their phone or half listening to you or distracted by their environment? Feeling undervalued is a common factor with many people I work with in my coaching/training business and sometimes the quickest way to alleviate this is to teach active listening. Do you ask the other person to put down their phone or eliminate distractions when you are talking to them or are you too concerned with offending someone? To practice this, spend one week really listening to other people not interrupting or giving your example of what they are talking about, just listen.. see what happens. Also, notice around you how many people half

listen to others, check out the body language, where are they looking, do they have their phone out? It is quite an eye opener when you people watch it can make you quickly aware of how you undervalue yourself and others. I love these two sayings "you never learn anything whilst you're talking" and "your ears never get you in trouble".

Have you ever met someone who gave you their full attention? What did that feel like? Give that gift to someone else.

20. A handy tip for developing rapport quicker with people is to repeat back some of their words to them. Not all of their words though as this may come across like mockery, when you use their words they feel familiar with you without knowing why. This also confirms with them that you are listening. People love to be listened to, don't you? Have you ever met anyone that you feel like you have known for ever, what was it about them that made you feel that? Was it the words they were using? Run it back through your head now and see if you can notice what made you

feel that?   Now spend the next 7 days playing with people's words, be aware of what you are saying and notice if you can build better relationships utilising this simple tool.

A smile can be seen from 100 m, what are you bringing to the party?

21. Did you know you cannot not communicate? You are continually giving out signals and pointers to those around you at an unconscious level through your body language. Just think about that for a moment, how do happy people move?   When someone is upset, how do they sit or stand? What do confident people exude through their physicality?   Everything from the gestures we make to the way we sit or stand sends out a message to those around us. What messages are you sending that you may not be aware of? What messages do you want to send?   One of the quickest ways to gain rapport with someone else is the match or mirror their body language. You already know how to do this, have you ever noticed people who are in love? They will mirror hand positions and head positions, friends do the same and when people feel comfortable with you

they tend to do the same. Spend some time noticing this around you and then see if you can build quicker and better relationships by subtly mirroring others. I say subtly because too much can be considered uncomfortable. Have a play with matching and mirroring and notice how others respond to you. People like people that are like us… just not too much.

"Tone of voice is the biggest indicator of a person's internal state"

22. Another way to gain rapport with someone quickly is to match their tone of voice and speed of speech. Again, if you make this too obvious it can become painful so use it with caution. Those small signals sent to the unconscious of the other person help them feel that you are familiar and this can lead to more effective communication and easier outcomes.

"Everybody has a unique map of reality. It is never about you"

23. Recognising that everyone is different and has a totally different soundtrack playing on their iPod can really help you relax in the company of others and appreciate your own uniqueness. When you think about people's perceptions in life take yourself back to the knowledge of how we process information and build our map of reality. All of our maps help guide us in life, if someone has an impoverished map they will judge everybody else based on their idea of what is right or wrong. This means that whatever someone says to you in the form of an opinion can never be about you. I know, that sounds weird but think about it, people judge based on what they would do, not what you are doing, so therefore it is never about you. This can take some contemplation to get the hang of but when you grasp this concept it makes it easy to allow others to have opinions without them ruining your day or making you feel anything.

"People tell you their internal state by the behaviours they show"

24. People are telling you their internal state when they talk. I always say "happy people don't cause problems" this is worth some consideration, how many happy people do you know that go around starting arguments or putting people down with negative comments? When someone is spitting fire at you it is worth remembering that they are showing you what they are feeling on the inside and do you really want to add to it. I think about it this way, I imagine that the person is my sister and if she was really angry or hurt what would I do? Would I shout back or would I walk off or would I listen, change my energy and bring her back to a better place? There are choices in every situation and not all people are self aware.. but you can be… it's just a choice.

"Assumptions make an ass out of me and you"

25. Never make an assumption, assumptions are the mother of all mess-ups. They also make an ass out of me and you. How often have you read a text and made a mind read that you know what the other persons intention was. Have you misread an email because you were feeling emotional and later found out that you took the wrong meaning from it. Have there been times when you have assumed that somebody had the hump with you only to find out they were experiencing issues elsewhere in life and it was nothing to do with you. How many times have you just sat down and made meaning of a communication with no solid evidence to back up the imagined thought process? What conversations have you had and then walked away from and run imaginary scenarios through your head about what you said, what you could of said or what meaning the other person took from the conversation? To avoid the unnecessary anxiety from the unknown factors just ask the question instead of assuming. Questions are the answer to everything, get curious and ask your life will become much simpler when you do.

"You are only aware of 3% of the 60,000 thoughts you have daily"

26. Pay attention to your thoughts they generate the state of being in your body. Spend 7 days just out of curiosity tuning in to the words that float through your mind. Are they supportive, motivating, debilitating, helpful, neutral, funny? Whatever you are thinking you will be feeling too. If you want to feel better, think better. Let those negative thoughts just drift through like clouds on a windy day and hold the positive thoughts in a space of contemplation to enhance the effect on the body. You think all day long, why not think yourself happy?

"Thoughts become things"

27. Thoughts become things, they are energy. Think of them like little signals that go out into the universe as indicators of what you want to experience in life. The more you think about something the more likely it is to appear in your life. What do you spend your time thinking about? Do you daydream about the things you

want to do in the future or what could possibly go wrong? Do you re-run old scenarios from the past re-experiencing all the negative aspects or do you reminisce on the good days and feel the joy, love, calm again? Everything in this world comes from thought first… from the pen to the sword without thought there would be nothing. I love that saying, it all begins in the mind first.

"Emotion is just energy in motion"

28. Your emotions are energy in motion. Knowing this means you can move them whenever you feel the need. Have you ever felt down and then done something and shifted the emotion, maybe you danced or listened to upbeat music or exercised or walked. It is all in your control, sometimes I like to hold negative emotions for a time as I think it is good to have balance (if you never feel bad how do you know what good feels like?) and then I move the feeling if it has lingered too long, my favourite is singing really loud to my dog, he loves it I'm sure :)

"Doing the same thing over and over expecting a different result is madness"

29. Have you ever heard the quote "The definition of mental illness is doing the same thing over and over again whilst expecting a different result?" If what you are doing is not working, try something different. What are you doing over and over in your life, whilst getting the same results (ones you don't want)? What could you change now that would free you up and release you from the grip of the loop you have been stuck in? Solutions come from trying a different approach. If you have a problem in your life now, what one small aspect could you change to start generating a solution? Change can be really uncomfortable and the majority of people like things to stay the same. Do you stay the same, moan and whine or make the change to shift the status quo? Remember you have choice, always.

"You deserve to succeed, raise your standards and expect more"

30. Raise your standards. You get what you expect. What do you expect in life, in relationships, in work, with friends? Do you expect to be successful or prosperous, happy or fulfilled? Have you even ever thought about your expectations? How have you created your current expectations? Are they based on the opinions of others throughout your life so far? Have you had an experience that has convinced you that you cannot create your dreams or that you do not deserve to achieve them? Spend some time writing down what you currently know about your expectations for yourself, be honest. Decide which ones of these are really working for you and then if you have some that are not working out, write down what you want instead, what would be your best outcome. You deserve to explore your full potential in life and by raising your expectations and standards you can start now.

"Your only limits are the ones you place on yourself"

31. Begin to remove your limitations. The only limitations we have in life are the ones we impose on ourselves. At what point did you stop dreaming? When we put ourselves in metaphorical boxes we stop exploring possibility and opportunity, this leads to stagnation and a lack of aspiration which can then lead to depression. We live in a world of labels and qualifications which for many people make them feel inadequate or undervalued, start exploring and becoming curious about what makes you tick, what lights your spark, what brings back that cheeky smile. Question the boxes that people have put you in and what you have labelled yourself with. How do you know all of these things to be true if you have never given it a go, what evidence is there that you cannot achieve your dreams if you really truly wanted to? Smash through the ceiling and start your journey.. for you.

"Reflect and learn, you are your own best teacher"

32. The mirror is an interesting concept, how much time do you spend reflecting on what you have done so far in life? When we are chasing goals people sometimes forget to reflect on the journey so far, full of twists and turns, bumps and hillocks, beautiful sunrises and stunning sunsets. What has got you to where you are today? What great qualities do you have that have helped you be the person you are now? What can you learn from your past self to have a better future? What did you do today that brings a smile to your face? If you could re-run the last week, what would you do differently to take you to the next level in your life experience? Reflect, daily, take the moments that will help you grow and sow the seeds for the brighter future you desire. The best lessons are the ones we take from ourselves, you are your best teacher when you view the past from the perspective of growth and opportunity.

*"You have earned it…
give yourself the credit
you deserve"*

33. Rewarding yourself for the small wins in life will increase your ability to motivate yourself. It doesn't have to be all about the big the goals and the rewards do not have to be massive. When you have achieved tasks throughout the day and reflected on what went well, reward yourself, have a hot bubble bath or watch a film, have a hot chocolate, read a book, take a walk, cook your favourite meal, just doing something with the intention of it being a reward for the jobs you got done throughout the day. It is a nice mental state to be in, knowing that you are getting something you really enjoy for achieving small goals.

"Take 10 minutes time out for you, no distraction, no phone, no email"

34. Taking daily time out for you should be the law. Many people spend so much time doing things for other people that they get to a point of burnout and overwhelm. To stop this happening designate specific blocks of time just for you. If you work for a company at least 10 minutes of your lunch break should be spent in your own thoughts, taking that well needed time out from the grind and resetting rebooting yourself for the rest of the day. The same in the evening, what time do you make for you? We all need that space to regenerate and relax, make sure you get yours.

"Get yourself in the mind gym. Your mind needs exercise just like the body"

35. How often do you exercise your mind as well as your body. What do you do in the mind gym? Have you ever considered this? Think of your mind like a muscle, if you don't use it there is a good chance it will drop into a state of atrophy. Learn something new each day, read a book, become curious about life, people, the world and allow your mind to grow. Every time we learn new information we create new connections in our brain this leads to expansion and growth. We become bored in life when we stop learning and growing… get yourself out of boredom, keep your mind learning so you can keep exploring your full potential.

"Great skin begins with hydration. Feeling tired? Drink water, you will be surprised by the results"

36. It is estimated that an adult body is between 55% & 65% water. Do you drink enough? The current school of thought is that you should drink a minimum of 2 litres of water a day. Water is vital to the body, if you feel thirsty you are already dehydrated. Start your body off in the right way in the morning, when you wake up drink a pint of water to replace the fluid you have missed out on whilst sleeping. It is recommend that you add something to the water you drink so it does not just go straight through you. My personal favourites are lemon and a pinch of himalayan rock salt. Once you get into the habit of drinking plenty of water you will notice the benefits in your body, less headaches, better skin, better body functions, less spots and less hunger. That is also one thing to consider, hunger and thirst are the same feeling so when you think you are hungry drink a small glass of water you may have just been thirsty.

"Kindness does not cost anything. How you treat others is a reflection of how you treat you"

37. Treat others as you wish to be treated yourself. You may have heard this many times when you were growing up. I did in my family, my parents always used this saying. My understanding of it now is that whatever you give out you get back. What does that mean to you? Do you spend your day angry at the world and find that you have interactions with angry people? Do you smile at strangers and notice how they smile back? I like to think of my emotional states and actions as gifts that I give to people, what gifts do you want to give out and receive? Spend some time noticing where your attention is when you are walking, driving or socialising, notice your state and how it affects others around you. Then look at other people interacting and become aware of what results they are getting and the process leading up to this. If we want something different in life we have to do something different.

"Not forgiving is the equivalent of wanting to poison someone else but drinking the poison yourself"

38. Forgiveness is one of the keys to happiness. How does it feel to hold a grudge against someone for years? Does it feel good to continually think about the wrong that person did to you? How much anxiety or anger or sadness or guilt do you run around the experience? Forgiving another human for their actions or words can free up your energy moving forwards. There is no need to actually speak to the person whom you wish to forgive, the act of picturing them in your mind and sending forgiveness to them will have the same effect. I do this regularly, not just with others but with myself too. It is a powerful emotion to let go of. How does it serve you holding onto the misgivings of others? What would be different in your life now if you just let it go? Write down a list of the people you wish to forgive and the reasons why this would benefit you, then send the forgiveness their way. I send it from the heart and as I do this I say to myself "I am sending this with love". Either let it go or let it eat you from the inside out… you have a choice.

"Be conscious of what you think because you get it"

39. Spend time with your thoughts. The majority of the time people just follow their thoughts blindly not noticing whether they are actually supporting them in life. Have you any idea what is running through your mind at the moment, we lose focus at least 20 times per minute and drift off into our head. Is it a good place to be? Take a moment to just stop now and become aware of the common thought streams you have, what do you spend most of the time thinking about? Jot down what pops up, good and bad, then decide if there is something different you want to think instead. Spending some time just listening to what you are running through your head can be a great way to filter out what you are wanting to experience in life. When you become aware of the percentage of negative vs positive thoughts you are having, try this, when a negative thought pops in your mind ask yourself if this is working for you, if not change it. Then when you have a supportive positive thought, hold it for a moment and enjoy the colours, the sounds, the feelings that come with it, maybe run it as a movie and play with the image for a while making it bigger and brighter. These habits of thought sifting will create a

happier state of being and develop the ability to focus on what you want out of life whilst sifting out the old past patterns.

"People are not what they do, they are what they believe to be"

40. All negative behaviour has a positive intention in some way. For someone to behave in any way it must serve them on some level. This is something that is taught to us early in life. If a child wants attention for doing good things yet is being ignored they will change their behaviour to negative to get a response, they want a response it doesn't matter to them if the response is good or bad its just attention. People who continually talk about their problems and how bad they feel about themselves tend to be surrounded by people who sympathise with them and tell them the opposite, this has a tendency to hold someone in the space of feeling bad not finding an internal solution to their inner feelings. Think of it like this, we have all seen those parents in the supermarket who have a screaming child demanding sweets and the parent said "no" 20 times whilst the child is still screaming and then

they get fed up and give in allowing the child the sweets. All this does is teach the child that if they want anything in life they just have to shout louder. What patterns do you have they may not be serving you to stand in the space of internal power? Do you seek attention, behave like a victim, rely on others, gossip, have negative self talk, withdraw alone, self medicate, receive financial handouts? The quickest way to develop yourself on a personal level is to grab life by the balls and find the power to rely on yourself. When you do this, you will find more balance and some inner peace.

"Finding the compassion for everything living will add to your daily sense of wellbeing"

41. Everything deserves kindness. Do you discriminate where your kindness goes? Do you love bees but hate wasps? Do you squash spiders but leave ants alone? This may sound like an odd learning however, having compassion and understanding for every living creature really does make you grateful to be alive. We have such a diverse mix of life forms on this planet yet

we spend so much of our day oblivious to the lives of these other species and dismiss them with a wave of the hand. What would change about your world view if you took some time to appreciate, not decimate the other species on this planet? Everything has a purpose, wasps eat insects, spiders eat flies, birds eat spiders. Just out of curiosity next time you go to swipe or squash, observe and become fascinated at the small or large life you are watching and appreciate it for the job it does here on the earth.

"Meditation means 'to become familiar with', take time to become familiar with you"

42. Discover a form of meditation that suits you. Being able to quieten the mind and focus your attention will aid your personal well being more than anything else. Meditation is not just about sitting cross legged making the sound "oohhm" it is about resting in the body, connecting back to nature and the universe, finding purpose, generating health in the body and creating the future how you want it to be. Meditation has been shown to reduce stress, control anxiety, promote

emotional health, enhance self awareness, lengthen attention span, reduce age related memory loss, lower blood pressure, generate kindness, help fight addictions and much more. Find something that works for you, relaxing music where you can daydream about your future, 10 minutes focused attention on your breathing, guided meditations, walking with purpose and attention to your surroundings, sitting in nature feeling gratitude. There are so many different ways to meditate and I recommend you explore as many as possible to find what suits you.

"Find common ground with others, make an effort"

43. Stop judging others, when you meet someone new ask them questions instead of checking out the clothes they are wearing or the car they pulled up in or the accent they have. We have been taught to judge everyone based on our own social upbringing this can be really limiting in life and you may be missing out on meeting some awesome people just through the pre-programmed judgements we make at a conscious and unconscious level. When you feel that little

tug in the body or hear yourself analyse another human being, ask yourself "what do I need to learn about myself to stop judging this person?". This is one of the quickest ways to grow and progress through life, take a learning from everyone about yourself.

"It's ok to ask for help. Successful people create this as a habit"

44. How often do you ask people for help? Do you sit in the space of overwhelm for days not daring to ask another soul for assistance or do you open up straight away? If you do not know the answer to something or how to do something, ask! Nobody knows everything and it is not a sign of weakness to ask someone else for their help or knowledge. Questions are the answer to everything. Is it worth your time and energy stressing yourself out for days or weeks over a subject that someone else could help you with? The older I get the more I ask for help, there is only so much I want to learn and if I do not have the knowledge and I know I can ask someone for assistance or guidance, I never hesitate nowadays. Through sharing knowledge we learn

and grow other peoples experiences can teach us so much, so drop the ego and get asking the questions to help you progress through life and business.

"Intuition is your guidance system, trust it. If it feels wrong, it probably is"

45. Trust your gut. We have an inbuilt guidance system that so many people ignore and if you follow it you will find more harmony and balance in life. How many times have you been asked to do something or go somewhere and it just felt wrong but you said yes? How often do you say yes to people when you really want to say no? I have a saying "wait a minute while I just run it through my system" what I mean by this is when I am asked if I want to do a job or go out somewhere, I check with my body first, does it get a hit of anxiety or do I feel mild excitement, do I get no response at all? If I feel the slightest bit of anxiety, I ask more questions about whatever it is someone wants me to do, if I still get a hit of anxiety I always say "no thank you". If my body gives me no response to the question I know that this means it will probably be ok or if I get a tinge

of excitement I definitely say yes. Your intuition will guide you when you listen. You all have it. Maybe you have just not been paying attention to it or have been ignoring it for years. I suggest tuning back in and experimenting with it. Spend some time 'running it through your system' and start trusting the responses you get. Maybe you will notice the changes in your life and your emotional state of being.

"We are meaning making machines, stop taking it all personally"

46. Take peoples words with a pinch of salt. Everybody has a different view on life and their view is no concern of yours. People can make suggestions and share opinions with you but it is only your decision that matters for your life. A great mentor of mine always said "it is one man's word" and this has probably been one of the most helpful learnings I have ever had. How do you know anything to be true? It is just one man's (or woman's) word. Check everything out yourself, do not fall into the trap of believing everything you hear. My grandad used to say "believe nothing of what you hear and only half of what you see", this

has stuck with me through the years and served me well. We have all heard of the game 'chinese whispers' information gets distorted when it is passed on and you never get the original version. People refer information differently based on their emotional state when they hear it and how they have been programmed in the past... remember the mind filters information at a phenomenal rate of knots. Our perceptual filters also alter what we see and we only see a small fraction of what is actually happening. Believe with a hint of curiosity as to the truth.

"Shine as an individual, never let another steal your light"

47. You are beneath no-one. You are more powerful than you know. Every breath you take is as worthy as anybody else on this planet. Find the value in you everyday. It doesn't matter how many degrees you have or certificates or companies you run, you are as valuable as the person stood next to you. We are taught that we have a lesser value than others at a very early age or we are taught that we have a greater value and develop a massive ego. No one has any

more right than anyone else on this planet. Spend some time now writing down and exploring the qualities that you have as an individual. What do you bring to this mixing pot of a planet? Stop comparing yourself to others and focus on you and your strengths in life.. we all have them.

"You are the creator of time, everything is now, be conscious of how you use it"

48. You are an island of time. If you could imagine being at sea in a beautiful sailing boat and in the distance you see an island, as you get closer to the island you notice it has 3 ports, the port of the past, the port of the present and the port of the future. You sail your boat straight into the port of the past and re-experience all of what has happened before then you sail your boat to the port of the present and spend some time in the now, finally you sail your boat to the port of the future and spend some time daydreaming about possibility and opportunity. After this you decide to get out of your boat and wander into the middle of the island where you discover there is a helipad, you jump in the helicopter waiting there and head straight up 200ft. From this space you

suddenly realise that you can see all 3 ports at the same time, you are never in the past because the past can only be accessed now, you are never in the future because the future can only be accessed now, you are only ever in the present as everything can only be accessed now. We do not get into a time machine and travel forwards or backwards, we only ever view it all now. So what are you bringing into the now? How much time do you spend re-living past drama? How much time do you spend future pacing yourself towards your dreams? How much time do you spend being in the now and enjoying the moment? Where do you gain most benefit..be curious.

"Slow down and pay attention to the small wonders of this world"

49. Enjoy the small things in life. The fact that you wake up and breathe so many people did not get that privilege today. Take time to notice the sky, the clouds, the rain and appreciate the beauty in how it continually changes. Listen to the birds and insects become familiar with their sounds and busy little lives. Appreciate your surroundings, the food you eat, the coffee/tea you drink, the

warmth of your home or the softness of your bed, there are people who have no bed or food or warmth. Enjoy the sunrise and the sunset they signal the beginning and end of another beautiful day. What small things do you have in your life that you can appreciate today? Do you have a job, a home, friends, food? Can you notice the complexity and beauty of this planet on your way to work? Are you aware of the simple kindness of other people when they smile or hold a door open? Opening up your awareness like this can help to lower levels of stress and find more peace on the inside. It also limits the continual chatter of the mind when it is being left unchecked to run its autopilot programs.

"You have the choice to make a difference. You get to choose your daily state of being, choose wisely"

50. Smile. A smile travels the world in a day. A smile can be seen from 100 metres away. A smile fills your body with the feel good chemicals that help the body heal. I challenge you to smile at least 50 times a day at anyone with a pulse. Raise your happy hormones and give others that little boost that might be the difference that made the difference. Maybe it was the only smile they saw today but you can make so much change in someone else by just changing the way you approach your day. Send out a love bomb and notice what you get back. In this universe of attraction and validation.. we get what we give out… what do you want in your life? What are you going to start giving now?

The best things in life are free!

Discovering You

Now that you have been on a brief journey of discovering you and how you operate as a system, let's take a look at how you can piece all of this information together to create a different way of being. It is fair to say that you should all now understand how every person on this planet has been preprogrammed by their environment, society, schooling, social engagements, tv, media and much more. Knowing this and becoming aware of how it benefits someone or not is the first place to start. So let us take a look at the programming so far.

Write down on the following 2 pages everything you know about your beliefs and behaviours so far, what you do, what you think, what you believe, what you perceive and then work out who or where did these pieces of information come in from. It is worth noting here that everything we know had to be taught to us. For someone to have a concept of colour, they had to be taught the colour spectrum. To have a concept of money, they had to be taught what money was, its value, its relevance and how it was to be used. To interact in a relationship they would have to have been taught the rules of engagement. Driving a car or riding a bike are both taught processes. So now you have an idea of the types of preprogrammed information that now generates behaviours, write your own list below. Many will be very beneficial yet some will be extremely limiting.

Example: I believe marriage is forever; society belief, parental belief.

I believe money doesn't grow on trees; parental saying, parents saved money, look after the pennies and the pounds will look after themselves.

I am not confident; comes from listening to other people and making comparisons between my success and theirs, teachers comparing me to others.

All people should be treated equally; parental belief because I grew up in a pub.

Success only comes from hard work; school belief, parental belief, media belief.

I am not good enough; childhood experiences, limiting teachers, unkind children at school.

I get angry really quickly; dad gets angry quick.

I am compassionate; mum is very compassionate.

I procrastinate; school teachers questioned me resulting in me not doing it quick enough.

People have to have university education to become millionaires; other people's beliefs.

Having this understanding of where we create our beliefs which leads to behaviours can be really beneficial when we want to change our life. You are currently the sum of everyone else around you until you become aware. Some people live the whole of their life never knowing anything other than their preprogrammed responses, is that where you want to be? Imagine waking up every day never knowing you have a choice to change the program, doing the same thing over and over wondering 'why' does this always happen to me? Just that process alone keeps the whole system turning doing the same thing time and time again, asking yourself 'why me' gives a signal to your system to find all the answers on the inside to validate the 'why me'. I always think what a beautiful supportive system we live in where whatever you ask it to do or think and it has to follow the command. How are you currently using your system? Are you giving instructions that are creating success or not?

"You have a choice to change the program"

It is estimated that 90-95% of your day is spent in autopilot mode. That means that you have habitual processes and ways of doing things that run at an unconscious level. This is a totally normal experience, everyone has it, the only problem is that some of the habitual processes may be very unhelpful and lead to unsuccessful outcomes. Your unconscious is the realm of operating systems, the reason we have them is to save time. Imagine having to learn everything again every time you woke up. Imagine having to name all the objects in your environment and create meaning for them all, you would never move off of the spot due to the overload of information. Think of it like this, you learn to tie your shoes through someone showing you and then practice, once you have learnt the information is then stored so you do not have to re-learn every time you want to put your shoes on, the same with driving, eating, socialising, walking, talking. You also do this with beliefs and emotions, if someone has experienced bullying early in life they now have a map for bullying. They may see bullying around them or take other people's comments personally and feel picked on in work or relationships. They could also have a belief system that they are worthless or not good enough or that something is wrong with them, this would then lead to behaviour attached to those belief systems.

So what did you discover when you wrote down your list of beliefs and behaviours above? Are there any things you do that are like your mum & dad? Can you see any patterns in your behaviour that stem from experiences you had in your early years or school?

Now I would like you to spend a few moments writing down the beliefs or behaviours you want to change and then let's look at a few ways you can change them.

What I would like to change.

One of the quickest ways to change a belief is to challenge it through questions. Byron Katie developed a series of questions to break apart the neurological boundary around a belief. A neurological boundary can be explained quite simply using the analogy of a balloon. If you imagine that the belief is inside the balloon and taking up space, through questions and resource adding we can pump positives into the balloon increasing its capacity until the balloon bursts, blowing the boundary around the problem or the belief. There are also ecology check questions and full brain posture or cross brain referencing to blow neurological boundaries, we will cover these below as well.

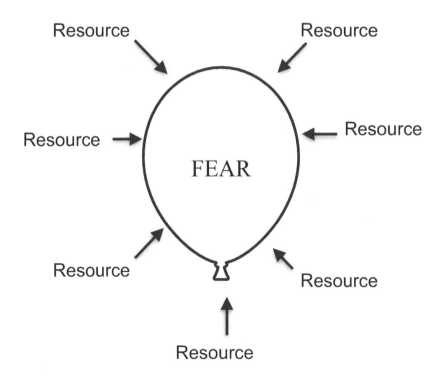

If you never know what is important to you in life then you may find yourself always walking down the wrong path and not feeling fulfilled or satisfied with where you are and what you are doing. Values, identity and beliefs are what we consider to be the top neurological levels for change which means that if a person is experiencing life in a space where they are not aligned to these aspects, then life may be very frustrating, depressing and hard work.

Transformation happens in someone's life when they shift on one of these levels. When that happens it creates a cascade effect on how they behave and access their knowledge, attitude and skill levels. Behaviour, knowledge, attitude and skill we call transactional processes and unless one of the top 3 levels of change have been experienced it can be really hard to maintain a new behaviour, develop a better attitude, access knowledge and utilise skill.

NEUROLOGICAL LEVELS FOR CHANGE

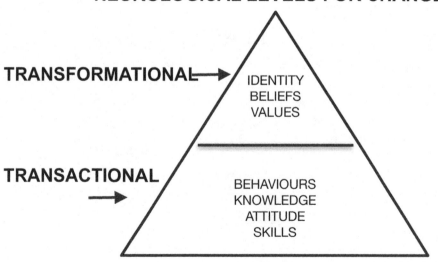

Discovering your values is a simple process. We just ask the question "What is important to you?". We want to give one word answers for this question and it is worth asking yourself this question around all areas of your life. Relationships, social life, health, business, recreation etc..

What is important to me about relationships? Here are some examples. The more you can write down the more fulfilment you will be able to experience in life.

Relationships: Trust, Honesty, Fun, Support

Work: Security, Fun, Appreciation, Trust

Social Life: Fun, Friendship, Community, Honesty

Now that you have a good idea about what is important to you in life, let us delve even deeper and find out your motivating factors that will help you succeed in all areas and find purpose and fulfilment. Ask yourself the following questions.

Why are these values important to me? What do they do for me, give me or get me? Here are some examples. The more you can write down the more fulfilment you will be able to experience in life.

Relationships: Trust, Honesty, Fun, Support.
Trust means I can feel safe and valued. Honesty means I can trust the other person and feel secure. Fun keeps me alive and I love laughing. Support means I can ask anything and get a truthful answer which leads to me feeling connected.

Health: Fitness, Strength, Diet, Sleep.
Fitness allows me to keep going through the day and feel good on the inside. Strength means I can take care of myself. Diet allows me to maintain a good weight and feel like I am looking after myself, I feel good when I eat well. Sleep is my reward for doing well in life, I sleep well when I am happy.

After we have discovered what is important to us in life and why, it is a good time to now check in and see if are values are being met in the different areas of life that you have listed above. Most people will find that if they are unhappy in a certain area of life it is because at some level their values are not being met. This can lead to unhappiness in relationships and total miscommunication, an easy fix would be if both couples did the exercise above and then found a way to fulfil the top 2 values of the other person.

This can be more difficult to fix in a working environment because the company structure, senior management, owners, directors or other staff members may be very inflexible in their attitude to change. It may mean leaving the company and pursuing a different working environment that suits the individuals needs.

Spend a few moments now looking at the areas of life you noted above and writing down what you are currently experiencing on the level of values in that space or place.

You will soon notice where you are getting fulfilment and having your values met and where there is room for improvement.

Work: Stress, Low morale, Lack of time.
Relationships: Fun, Friendship, Lack of time.
Health: Fitness, Strength, Tiredness.

So what are you now noticing about your life? How happy and fulfilled are you? Are you beginning to notice how some beliefs may be holding you back and how in some areas of life your values are not being met?

You should also be realising by now that you have some really good beliefs too and that there are aspects of your life that are going really well.

The final aspect of neurological levels for change is identity, who you think you are? Most people find after doing the following exercises that they are not who they think they were in the first place. Let me give you a scenario to think about first so you can begin to unravel the mystery of you.

Imagine you are just entering a multi screen cinema and there are 100's of movies available for you to watch, you read through all of the film titles and decide that the first movie you are going to see is 'the movie of me'. You walk into the cinema and sit down and the movie begins, you notice that this really is 'your' movie, you know all of the characters, your mum, dad, sister, brother, friends, colleagues and it all feels really familiar. You are exactly as you know you to be.

Then you walk out of this cinema and head for the next screen. This is the movie of your mum. As the film starts you begin wondering who the woman is on the screen because she talks differently to how you know her, she behaves differently, she even looks slightly different to how you know her. You notice that when she speaks about you, you do not recognise who she is talking about. It occurs to you that her perspective of everyone around her including yourself, is totally different from what you thought it should be.

The next movie you go into is the movie of 'your dad', again the same thing happens you begin to wonder who this person is, they are not acting how you know them to be. The perspective they have of themselves is totally the polar opposite to your perspective of them. Now you are getting confused, so you go to watch your best friends movie and guess what? Yes, you have guessed it, they have a totally different perspective of you to your parents, sister, colleagues and your own perspective. So you now think to yourself "I am going back to the movie I know, me".

When you walk back into your own movie theatre you realise that you are now not that sure who the person on the screen actually is. You begin to question what you thought you knew about yourself. You begin to question everything you know about you and all of the perspectives of other people. Who are you?

The purpose of this scenario is to allow you to explore what you think you know about yourself and view yourself from multiple perspectives. You may find that you act a certain way around particular people and then totally different around other individuals. What I would like you to explore is how you get to this point, where did you learn to be a certain way? Do you like the person you are in all of these situations?

What do you love about you?

What behaviours do you like that you do?

What qualities do you have?

What are your strengths?

What do you not like about you?

What behaviours do you not like that you do?

What qualities do you not like?

What are your weaknesses?

Now with all of the above I would like you to allow yourself to wander down the list and make a note of where and from whom do you think you learnt how to do these things. This is just to raise your awareness of how everyone is programmed with the knowledge of how to function in life. For you to operate on a daily basis, remember we need to have a map to the future and this map is created throughout our early years. This process also continues into adulthood, we are always learning.

Consider this question now, who are you when you are experiencing the positive feelings and emotions? To begin to find the authentic version of who you want to be, notice the behaviours you run when you are happy or relaxed. Who do you believe yourself to be at those times? What are the 'I am' statements attached to those states of being?

I am content

I am happy

I am a good person

I am at peace

I am successful

What you will begin to become aware of is that when you are in certain states of being, are running particular emotions or feelings, you will be more productive, energetic or motivated. For those of you wanting to create more success in your businesses, knowing what states generate the levels of performance needed for you to achieve your goals is essential because if you are functioning in the lower levels of emotions or feelings, then you are limiting your personal performance which can affect your business. The same goes for relationships or health or sport, the state we are in has a massive effect on the outcome we achieve. Utilise the belief busters below to check in that your 'I am' statements are true and felt on every level. For someone to move forwards and create success in life they have to believe congruently throughout their system that it is possible. Any doubt can seriously slow down the process. When we remove doubt the universe tends to flow through us unrestricted and possibilities and opportunities appear as if by magic. When people experience the state of flow they tend to have no problem at all manifesting their desires and goals. Your aim through the following processes is to get your system into the state of flow as often as possible and remove barriers and blocks that are limiting you in life. My suggestion would be that you start with the negative beliefs that are the least resistant, begin with the smallest chunks first and then when you reach the big ones they will have much less weight in them and the process will be easier.

Belief Busting

There are 2 main stages to creating beliefs, opinion and re-enforcement. Opinions are surrounding us all day long, people love to share an opinion and they will always have one about the majority of decisions you are about to make or things you want to do. You will also have masses of opinions about other people and yourself. This is totally normal as we all have our own map of reality and each of our maps is totally unique and different to everyone else's. Remember that people can only judge any situation by their own previous experiences, fears, limitations and emotions. To some people starting their own business would be an exciting journey, yet for someone else it would be filled with terror and you have to wonder how they became programmed to think that working for yourself is terrifying, someone had to install the doubt somewhere. Once we have listened to an opinion from ourselves or another, we then contemplate it and this is the re-enforcement aspect. The more we question ourselves and add conviction to the negative comment/opinion then the more we begin to install a belief that will start to generate a specific type of behaviour. Do you really need to listen to opinions? I would suggest you create a habit of laughing at yourself on the inside when you hear an opinion and asking yourself the question "Is this helpful?", if the answer is yes, then contemplate that particular opinion until it becomes a supportive belief, if the answer is no, then let it go over your head like a Giraffe's fart and drift off into the distance never to be thought again.

The first belief busting tool I am going to share with you was created by Byron Katie. This amazing lady had spent the first 40 years of her life depressed and overweight, she checked herself into a rehab unit and whilst in there had an epiphany. This led to her developing the 4 questions you are about to learn and totally transforming her life. She realised that nothing was real or true and this opened her up to become free from the self imposed limitations we all have. Utilise these questions to pull apart your beliefs and find some freedom from those restrictions.

Example of belief: I will never be successful.

1. Is it true? (Yes or no. If no, move to question 3.)
2. Can you absolutely know that it's true? (Yes or no.)
3. How do you react, what happens, when you believe that thought?
4. Who or what would you be without the thought?

Turn the thought around. I will be successful. I will succeed. People succeed so I can. Success is easy.

Now spend a moment visualising what success looks like and contemplate each one of the statements noticing what it looks like, feels like and sounds like to be the new belief.

These questions work by challenging the structure of the belief and its validation. When we use questions to unpick the truth, the neurological boundary around the problem belief is blown and this then leaves you in a space to install a new more functional productive belief.

Recent neuro-scientific studies have shown that it takes around **72 hours** to install a new belief. We have a saying amongst the people I work with and that is "only clean the teeth you want to keep". If you think of your thoughts and beliefs like teeth, which ones do you want to keep shiny and clean and which ones do you want to die away. Whatever we give our attention to will keep showing up in our lives, so instead of being aware of what you are thinking, be conscious of what you are thinking because your thoughts become things.

The second belief busting tool is something I call cross brain referencing. This involves crossing hands and feet simultaneously which in turn fires up both hemispheres of the brain. This one takes patience and practice. Firstly, decide on the belief you wish to change, then find a nice quiet space where you can sit undisturbed for at least 5 minutes. Sit down and cross your ankles and your wrists, close your eyes and begin repeating the new belief that you want to have whilst allowing in all the negative thoughts that hold you in the space of the old belief. This is very important that you do not push away the negative, just allow it to flow through you as you continually repeat out loud the new belief. You will notice that at some point during the 5 minutes certain things will happen, you may feel a shift in your breathing or a sense of well being or you will just hear the negative thoughts stop and all that is left is the repetition of the positive belief. Remember again to repeat this process a good few times over the next 72 hours to ensure that the new belief is fully installed.

Now let us take a look at Socratic questioning, this was used by Socrates to change and challenge beliefs. It is based on the principle of 'the meaning you give an event is the belief that attracted it'. Think about this for a moment, if someone held a belief that no-one liked them how do you think they would perceive group interactions? Would they be perceiving them as places where everyone talks to them or would they be seeing the situations where they are alone in the room or not fitting in? We are meaning making machines and our perception of events can have a powerful impact on our life. Contemplate for a moment the opposite belief, that they were a likeable person, how would that feel different? Try them both on for size so you can get a feel of those 2 perceptual beliefs. Which one do you prefer?

Once again, pick a belief that you wish to change and run yourself through these questions. It is really important that you write down your answers as this allows you to be really objective, get it out of your head and onto some paper.

Example belief: I can never be happy

1. Do you believe that?
2. Why do you believe that?
3. What do you prefer to believe instead?

Do not judge your answers, just allow yourself to be an observer and use the questions to guide you to an alternative.

It is worth remembering that beliefs are not facts they are thoughts that became re-enforced by social development, peer programming and self analysis. Beliefs and facts are totally different. Beliefs are a thought we have faith in and facts are something that is proven to be true. Many people hold total faith in their negative beliefs which leads them to lead a life of quiet desolation. To gain more from your life experience becoming aware of and clearing out limiting beliefs is the best place to start because your beliefs generate all of your behaviours. Be open and willing to go against your natural flow of thought and experience something new.

There is an interesting way of clearing beliefs that was developed in Hawaii by Morrnah Nalamaku Simeona it incorporates a practice of reconciliation and forgiveness. This idea behind this is that you clear yourself to help clear the world. The 4 statements are said on the inside (not out loud) and are used to dissipate and clear negative emotions or feelings which are hidden beliefs. When people feel bad about something it tends to be linked to an unconscious belief system and the people of Hawaii use this process to cleanse themselves and the mirror self of those around them. Have you ever heard the phrase 'they are your mirror"? You can only recognise in others what you have within you. If you spend time considering your emotional responses to other people and their actions you will notice that deep down you have a belief linked to these and because of the understanding of the universal field theory stating that all is energy and everything is intrinsically linked to the next, this would make sense that through clearing your own negative emotional connections you will benefit the field in general.

Use this process when you experience a negative emotion or feeling (you must be feeling it), whatever you can feel you can heal. When you feel the negative emotion or feeling repeat the following statements internally, in any order you want until the emotion disappears.

1. Thank you
2. Please forgive me
3. I'm sorry
4. I love you

I have found this very effective for removing the negative emotions and hidden beliefs because I am quite connected to how I feel. This has been a quick peaceful process for me to follow and I use it daily. Allow yourself to sit with and not try to rush the process. Think of this like a combination lock that unlocks a clearing space where new supportive beliefs can be born.

It is worth noting here that the new beliefs you want to experience should be fitting with your life expectations. They need to be congruent with your system in its present state of being. What I mean by this is that if you are wanting something that carries masses of emotional weight and you are constantly fighting yourself to clear the emotions, you may need to start from a gentle place with very little resistance. Think of this like peeling off layers of an onion, you cannot get to the core before you have unwrapped the outside layers. Be patient!

"To peel an onion, you have to start from the outside layers and work inwards. You cannot unwrap the core first "

Trigger Driver Behaviour

For you to create success in all areas of your life it is important to understand the following principles that apply to everything we do. As you are now aware, you are preprogrammed with autopilot responses that save time and allow you to function on a daily basis in all situations. Awareness is one of the greatest tools to changing how we behave. When you become aware of what triggers you, you can get a head start on changing the emotions and behaviours that are the end result of the trigger. Triggers are normally something you hear, see, feel, say to yourself or do. Memories can be triggers, people, smells, tv shows, songs, colours, words, they are all around us all of the time.

Let us look at a case of PTSD to help make sense of this process. Imagine someone has experienced a high speed motorbike crash which left them with debilitating injuries. Previous to their accident they had no issue seeing or hearing loud motorbikes and they were probably quite happy driving at speed. The emotional trauma embedded during the accident would have set into motion some interesting behavioural responses that at an unconscious level have been developed to keep the person safe. What they might experience is a response to seeing bikes travelling past at high speed or if they see them on the tv or even hearing them in the distance. The response they may experience could be panic or anxiety or fear. The resulting emotion will then create a behavioural response which could be quite negative. This could be anything from a physical internal response i.e. shaking or feeling sick to an external response of running or lashing out in some way.

Think about someone being bullied at school. The process of bullying would have created numerous negative emotional states within the person leading to behavioural responses. Imagine the effect of this later in life, the bullied person would then have a map of how to behave when they experience triggers. They may perceive that they are being bullied when someone raises their voice or changes their facial expression. They may read something that would trigger a negative emotional response. Their perspective would be filtered through the lease of bullying.

We do not just have triggers for negative experiences, we have triggers for everything. How would you know you were thirsty? Would you feel something, see something, say something to yourself or hear something? There has to be a start point (trigger) for you to know you want a drink. Think of being happy, how would you know it is time to be happy? Would it be someone you saw or something you heard?

When we become aware that we have triggers firing off all day long then we can begin to change our responses to them. If we know that certain things fire us up and allow us to generate a particular behavioural response it means we can be prepared for situations and give ourselves an option to change how we behave. How we respond to something is actually a choice that we make, however, because it happens so quickly it can take us by surprise. Knowing this means that we can take a look back at situations that have not turned out great and analyse the triggers that created the driving emotions which led to the non adaptive behaviour. Hind sight is a great tool that when utilised can help us change in the now, the responses we demonstrated before.

The emotions generated in every moment drive the behavioural response. When we know that a certain situation is a trigger for a negative emotion, we can prepare ourselves to generate a different emotional state at that time which will alter the behaviour.

Emotions are the driver and emotions are just energy in motion.   It is a moving feeling that can be manipulated and moved into something else or just observed and allowed to pass by. People do not have to act on their emotions, they can just observe them yet so many of us respond instantly to the feeling without even checking in if it is going to be beneficial to us.

Just consider now for a moment how many times you have been triggered into emotional responses. Are there certain songs you hear that bring a smile to your face or a rush of energy into your body? Are there certain people that you know who when you think about them or see them you just feel good? Do you have certain words that people say to you that instantly fire that negative energy within you?

In the training environment where I spend the majority of my time, we use something called an adaption model.   This model helps to raise awareness of your triggers and allows you to begin to develop different responses and gain control over the habitual processes that your unconscious runs when triggered.

On the next page let's take a look at what you know about your current life triggers and the emotions and behaviours you run in these situations.

Positive Triggers	Emotion	Behaviour - End Result
Tina Turner Simply the Best	Happiness	Singing and Smiling - Feeling Good

"You are not what you do, you are what you believe on the inside"

Negative Triggers	Emotion	Behaviour - End Result
The News	Frustration	Turning TV Off

"Change is a choice, choose a different result"

What did you notice from the exercise? Has it raised your awareness to the small things that you become reactive to? How many times a day do you get triggered by small experiences that then generate an over reactive result?

The start point to being able to react less is to become aware first. Knowing that certain situations or people allow us to create chemical reactions in our body that lead to non productive behaviours means that we can prepare prior to the majority of events.

How many ways do you know already that can change your state of being? What do you currently do to alter the way you feel?

I Change My State By:

Turning TV Off

Listening to Music

Dancing

Now you have listed all of the ways you can change your state, think about which ones are suitable for which situations so you can prime yourself with a better start point before the events/people/places/sounds/memories that trigger you.

Negative Triggers	Emotion	Positive Action or Solution
The News	Frustration	Turning TV Off
A Certain Person	Anger	Decide to Not React - Think about Favourite Holiday - Breathe Deeply and Smile Inside
Upcoming Presentation	Fear	Tina Turner in the Car

With the whole of this book, it is the doing that will make a difference. Many learn skills and search for knowledge yet never apply it. The more you develop your skills and tools around changing your state on demand, the happier you will be in life. The less you give your brain control by allowing it to run the autopilot programs that you have developed over the years, the more balanced and stable your life will become.

These skills and techniques take practice, practice does not make perfect, it makes permanent!

Remember the saying "only brush the teeth you want to keep", this is relevant to the whole of your life in every area. Whatever you nurture and give your attention to will grow and flourish. This means all of the negative as well as all of the positive. So what is it that you want to grow?

No one can affect change in your life except you! Owning every aspect of your being will allow you to become powerful beyond measure. It will allow you to create the impossible (I'm-possible). You will notice that your thought process slows down and that little voice in your head becomes quieter and quieter until you have mind peace. You may still have the odd negative thought pop up but it will be so obvious that you can just grab it and challenge it there and then.

"Practice does not make perfect, it makes permanent"

Ownership

This is one of the toughest things to do in life because we are taught to blame everyone else for our situations and make up reasons or excuses for why things did not happen in our lives or why we are unable to do something.

"There wasn't enough money"
"I lived in the wrong area"
"No one in my family ever went to University"
"The teacher didn't like me"
"I'm not good enough to succeed"
"I can't try"
"I am just an angry person"
"They don't make me happy"
"No one supports me"

We seem to live in a world where people share their pain points with each other, it is like some weird bonding ritual where we share pain and then try to out do each other with more pain.

Spend some time listening to other people talk and notice how many excuses/reasons people come up with to avoid situations or self ownership and how many pain conversations do they have. An example would be someone complaining about a bad back and then their friend say's "oh yes, well my hip was killing me yesterday". It will amuse you and disappoint you at the same time when you realise that you are a pain sharer too. Raising your awareness around the pain sharing aspects of our society will allow you to bring more balance and peace to your daily environment and also to those around you. Remember that your brain is like google, give it a rubbish question and it will give you a rubbish answer, whatever you put in comes out. So, if you are spending your day sharing pain points and making excuses or creating reasons to not do things, are you going to be feeling good and positive?

Awareness is the best tool you can ever have in your toolbox of life. Most people just float through life following their autopilot responses and never become aware of the continual negative patterns that are running and causing them to feel down.

We come across extremes of this when we work with people who have intense road rage. They are continually blaming other road users for their internal state and behave in a fashion that is increasing their levels of negative bio chemistry and actually making them ill. They seem to have lost the ability to rationalise the facts that no one is perfect and everyone makes mistakes whilst driving, they do too. Yet when they get into the state of rage it has to play itself out to the end, sometimes with extremely negative results that last for weeks. They hold the state for as long as they possibly can, which is interesting because it is the equivalent of self punishment. They seem to have lost all control over their thought processes and self instigated responses.

When you become aware of these overwhelming experiences that can create such damage outside and inside, you get to choose a different response. The simplest way to generate instant change is just to take a deep breath and say something like "well that's interesting" on the inside and then smile, remind yourself that no one is perfect and everyone makes mistakes. This does take lots of practice and if someone has had many negative experiences in their life they may have so much stored negative emotion that they find this a massive challenge. There are numerous ways to recode and remove stored emotion and I recommend researching some of these if you know anyone who continually has problems with emotional overload (I will make notes in the end of the book).

Take a moment to note down what you do not own in your life. Where do you put blame or expect someone else to supply the outcome for you? Notice where you make excuses and use reasons to not engage.

What Do I NOT Own:

My Happiness

My Ability to Learn

My Anger

My Life Choices

Ownership = Power, when you take back ownership of your emotions, life choices, beliefs and behaviours, you can really create great change in your life. It is an empowering experience to acknowledge what you have control over. No one ever gets to dictate your emotional states to you or discourage you with their opinions. You will stop comparing yourself to other people and start following your own path in life.

What would your life be like now if you took full ownership, what would change for you? Would your weight change or your physical appearance? Would your circle of friends change or your working environment? Would you leave the relationship that is not working or would it strengthen it? Would you still be living in the same house or would you move to where you have always wanted to be? Where would you be spending the majority of your time and with whom?

It is interesting when we look at our lives through a full state of open ownership, this gives us the opportunity to filter through what we really want in life that allows us to generate that true inner happiness and sense of control.

Becoming aware and owning our lives opens us up to a new source of energy and a sense of self. You will find you have more motivation to achieve even the smallest of things. You will find your attitude changes and when this happens, the world is your oyster.

"Ownership = Power. Take back control and open up to endless possibility"

Yes

Did you know that the universe only ever says yes to you? Did you know that your human system is designed to only ever say yes to you?

What a strange thought that we live in a dimension that only ever says yes and that our human system is built to do the same. Consider it for a moment. Have you ever heard of the Law of Attraction, this is a believed law that governs the whole universe. The basics of it are that like attracts like. What ever you are thinking about or feeling you will be attracting into your life. Just think about that for a moment and see if it is true for you. The best way to understand these laws and make a decision is to become totally honest with ourselves and try it on for size. Denial (not the river in Egypt) is a desolate space where no growth can take place. Use the space below to note down your current and previous life experiences, thoughts, beliefs and feelings and pay attention to them with relevance to the Law of Attraction.

Event	Emotion/ Belief	Result
Didn't Like School	Sadness, Anger	Numerous Experiences of Bullying, Negative Teachers and Bad Results
First Kiss	Excitement	He Kissed Me Out of the Blue
Rough Relationships	Didn't Deserve Better	Unhappy Relationships

So what did you notice, have you attracted what you have in your life or did you take a trip down the river of denial?

Pay close attention to the emotions and thoughts you were having when you attracted those positive aspects into your life, this is your guidance system giving you some really good pointers of what works. Then also pay attention to the emotions or thoughts you were having when you got a negative result, this is also a great pointer to how to not get stuff to work in your life.

The system you walk around in is designed to support you in life and get you all of the results that you ask for. It is a validation system. This system has been preprogrammed for you through childhood so you have a good map of how to function everyday of your life in every situation. Think about that for a moment. Who taught you to do money, relationships, health, importance of study or not, friendships, values, beliefs, compassion, anger, guilt, happiness? All of these aspects and more are taught to us in some way shape or form in our younger years, just like we are taught to tie our shoes or use a knife and fork, we are taught emotions and beliefs about possibility, opportunity or not. How limited have you been in life and not known why? Start asking yourself the questions of where did I learn that limitation or negative belief about myself/life? When you become more aware of this process, you can unlock your future and free yourself from the past. It is worth remembering that if the past goes unchecked it creates habitual autopilot programs that run continually to save us time, it is being as helpful as it possibly can. Your mind (conscious & unconscious) have an integral part to play in your auto pilot programs, your whole system is helping you out so you do not have to re-learn everything everyday. Whatever you do not check in on, challenge or change will consistently run for you. Your system wants to help, it only ever says yes!

"Yes you are good enough"
"Yes you are not good enough"
"Yes no one likes you"
"Yes most people like you"
"Yes you can succeed"
"Yes you can't succeed"

There are certain parts of your brain that spend their whole time looking for what you are focusing on. Imagine that, you actually have tools in your head like mini radars that scan your environment for what you are thinking or believing at any time! This process takes place because your conscious brain has limited processing space per second compared to the unconscious, so it has to be very particular about what it filters and what it makes you aware of.

My Current Aspects of Focus are:

Peace

Generating More Clients

Worrying About Money

Worrying About Work

Having Fun

Being Happy

People's Opinions

Now write yourself a 'Yes' list that you really want to experience in your everyday life. Go into plenty of detail and use the belief busting tools to remove any negativity that may arise when you think about what you would really want to experience.

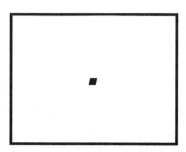

Imagine this box is your whole day and the dot is your point of focus for the day…. what are you focused on? You could be missing some amazing stuff … change your focus change your future!

"Thoughts become things, be conscious of what you are thinking"

Energy

Are you aware that you are an energy being? Are you aware that you have an electro magnetic field surrounding you that connects to the planet? Do you know that every cell in your body generates energy and that the average human, in a state of rest generates 100 kw of energy. You are basically a walking power station converting energy from different sources and utilising this for multiple functions in the body. The relevance of knowing this is that you only have a limited source of energy everyday to use and you can deplete this source really quickly if you are unaware of this.

I like to think of energy generation coming from two main sources, our food and our environment. So let us take a look at the environment first.

Have you ever been in a place where you just feel like the energy is being drained out of you? Maybe the place you work, or a social setting. Have you ever had that feeling of walking into somewhere and literally feeling the good vibes being drained out of your system? Was it a certain person or multiple people or was it the actually ambience in the building? I like to call this being 'mood hoovered' because it is like someone has turned on a high powered vacuum and is sucking the life out of you. You must have also had those experiences where you walk into somewhere and you feel energised, what was it about that environment? Was it the colours, the people, the sounds, the smells? Did you notice in that space that you felt more alert, energised and responsive?

"Beware of the Mood Hoovers"

Just try this simple exercise for a moment so you can begin to realise that even thinking about events can give you responses. Think of a time when you went somewhere and felt like you were being mood hoovered, drop right back into that moment and allow yourself to feel what your body feels like when it is a negative space. Do you notice it via sensations in the body or thoughts or through your breathing? Now think of a time when you went somewhere that totally energised you and made you feel great. Check in with the body as you recall the event and again notice where you feel those feelings or sensations, how do you sit or stand differently, what thoughts are you thinking. Did you notice the difference? Were the pictures you created in your mind different? Were the happy ones colour and moving or framed and still? Were the negative ones black and white, small and dark? The more you pay attention you will realise that our brain works in pictures and creates images based on the emotions we feel, so if you want to feel better in a negative space a quick tip is to change the pictures in your mind to brighter more colourful images.

Now let us take a look at how our thoughts can drain us or juice us up. The arrows pointing out signify energy being drained from us, the arrows pointing in signify energy coming back to us.

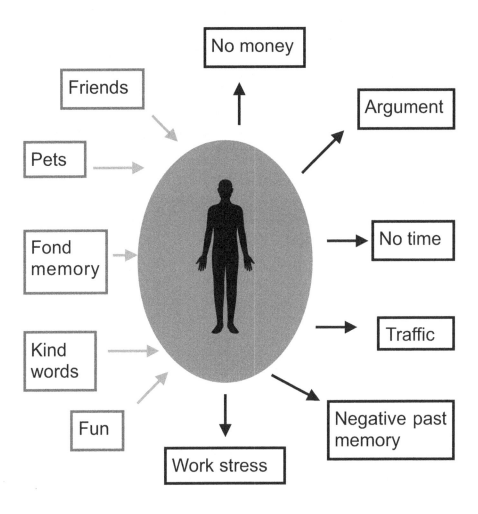

Every exchange you have on a daily basis will either feed your energy or deplete it. What are your main areas of focus? Did you know it is estimated that we have around 60,000 thoughts a day and we are only aware of about 3-5% of those. Can you imagine what you are thinking at an unaware level that is draining your energy or juicing you up? It can be quite a scary thought. If you imagine every thought you send out is money and you either get a return on your money or lose it. When you put your focused attention on the negative you lose money, however when you put your attention into the positive you get a 100% return on your money. Would you purposefully give something you disliked a large sum

Just spend a few moments jotting down below some of your current energy expenditures via thoughts and interactions with others and write down if they are working for you or not.

Subject	Time Spent	End Result - Juiced or Drained

What did you notice? How much energy are you expending on negative interactions of thought or experience, how much are you regaining from positives exchanges?

If there is a big gap then maybe it is time you took a look at your environment to find out where you need to make the changes that will create the biggest shift in life for you.

My experience over the years has shown me to keep balance. It is ridiculous to think that you can avoid all negative interactions in life because most external things are out of your control, however, you can limit your exposure to them and this is what I do on a daily basis.

I do not watch the news on the tv, listen to the news on the radio, watch reality tv or soap operas, spend time with negative people, allow myself to sit in victim mentality. I make a choice to limit the amount of negativity coming in so I can achieve a state of balance. If I am running at 80% good 20% not so good, then I find my days/weeks/months and years are pretty productive and happy. Find the balance that suits you so you can experience more positive emotions and balance in your life.

The second main source of energy is food. This is so simple to keep in balance when you just listen to your body. The majority of people are habitual eaters, they eat breakfast lunch and dinner at set times whether they are hungry or not. This is mass pre-programming on a global scale. We do not need to eat half the food we currently eat. Have you noticed if you are ever actually hungry before you eat? Is it just a habit? Do you know that your stomach is the size of your fist and you should put no more food than that on your plate? Are you programmed to finish every morsel or do you stop eating when you no longer feel hungry? Do you check if you are hungry or thirsty before you eat because hunger and thirst feel the same? If you are habitually eating and not feeling hungry you are continually filling up a tank that is already full. Would you do that to your car? If you tried to fill up your petrol tank when it was already full, the petrol would spill onto the floor, a total waste of fuel, this is the same for the body apart from it doesn't spill onto the floor, it turns into fat.

Here are some tips to help your body generate energy and for you to find your natural balanced weight and stay there with no effort.

1. Only eat when you are hungry. Measure the hunger on a 1-10, when you hit 5/6 eat.
2. Avoid eating after 7pm in the evening. Allow your body time to digest and repair you.
3. Only eat breakfast if you are truly hungry. It is only the most important meal of the day if you are hungry, otherwise you are just storing fat.
4. Control your portions to the size of your fist. Eat slower and stop when you no longer feel hungry.
5. Drink 2 litres of water with lemon oil or lime oil per day. The oil will help create an alkaline environment in your body and helps the water to

be absorbed efficiently rather than just go straight through you. I recommend a good quality oil like Do'Terra. Something natural with no additives.
6. Choose organic food as much as possible.
7. Avoid pre packed meals.
8. Look after your gut health as this is intrinsically linked to emotional health. (see back of book for recommendations).
9. 20-30 minutes exercise 3-5 times a week. Choose the stairs instead of the lift, get off the bus 2 stops early, make a choice to move more often because movement generates energy.

For the past 25 years I have remained the same weight and have always eaten in a particular way. My day starts with a pint of water and a cup of coffee, I have a snack at between 12-2 which would consist of a piece of fruit or some peanut butter on dates, then I eat early evening if I feel hungry (sometimes I don't because I have not expelled enough physical energy) my meal would be proteins and veg. Every now and then I like a sweet treat however this is quite rare because I just don't feel the need, my body gets its sugar from the dates and fruit. If I want something sweet after dinner, I eat less dinner to accommodate the sweet. The point is to become aware of when you are overeating due to habits and overfeeding due to portion size or beliefs around wasting food. It is also worth noting that when people have a lot of stored up negative emotion they tend to overeat. Remember this is about finding something that works for you, there is no one size fits all. Current studies of eastern traditions show that intermittent fasting is a great way to keep the body healthy and clean. This is basically 16 hours of no food with an 8 hour eating window. Basically the equivalent of what I do.

Try it and just notice how different you feel.

"What you believe about food, you will be"

What Will You Do NOW?

Unless you have a plan moving forwards it is unlikely that you will reach your goals. There have been many studies over the years based around planning for the future or goal setting. It has been shown on numerous occasions that people who write down their goals for the future are more likely to achieve them than people who don't. Think of your brain like a sat-nav that needs a destination inputed so it knows where it is going. If you wanted to drive from Devon to Scotland and you did not look at a map or set a destination in your sat-nav you could end up anywhere and may takes you years to randomly hit your destination. Your brain needs direction and it does not matter how many times you adjust the route, as long as you at least give it a starting direction.

I like this analogy for setting a direction; If you wanted to go home after a night out and ordered a cab, then instructed the driver to "not take me to the library", where would you end up? If the driver did not know where you lived, where would they take you? You could end up anywhere and it would be very unlikely they would find your house. So make sure you set a clear direction. Give specific instructions, not wishy washy unclear coordinates.

If you wanted more money, what would that amount be? Not setting a clear amount could result in you finding 1p on the floor…. there you go, more money!

So what would more money look like? Is it a wage increase from £25k per year to £45k per year? Is it a monthly income or a weekly income? Is it a to have £6 million in the bank? What specifically do you want? The more specific you get the more your brain has to focus on finding for you. I recommend that you do this process starting with a 10 year goal and break it backwards into to sections. The reason is because most people do not have an end state, that ultimate destination that draws them forwards. Ask yourself what it is that will ultimately fulfil you in life? Then back step with a 7 year goal, 5 year goal, 3 year goal, 1 year goal, 9 month goal, 6 month goal, 3 month goal and 2 week goal. Doing this will create your master map for your future and keep you on track when you wander.

Imagine someone wanting to feel more happiness in their life, what would that look like, feel like, sound like? What would they be doing and thinking on a daily basis to have this feeling on the inside? Where would they be going? Who would they be associating with?

Remember that you are the creator of your map of reality, the more detail it has the easier it is to navigate your way around it. So let's look at some ways of filling in your map so you have a really good image and landscape to follow.

What specifically do you want?

Why do you want this?

Where are you now in relation to the outcome on a scale of 1-10?

What will you see when you have achieved this goal?

What will you hear when you have achieved this goal?

What will you feel when you have achieved this goal?

What will you be saying to yourself when you have achieved this goal?

What are the main steps that will let you know you are achieving this goal?

What will this outcome get for you or allow you to do?

Is it only for you and are you prepared to take full ownership of the goal?

Where and when do you want to achieve this goal?

How do you want to achieve this and with whom?

What do you have now to help you achieve your goal?

What do you need to get to achieve your goal?

Have you ever had or done this before?

Do you know anyone who has achieved this and what can you model from them?

What behaviours have held you back in the past?

Imagine yourself in the future now, what behaviours will you change to achieve your goal?

When will you start doing these?

What will you gain when you achieve your goal?

What will you lose if you don't achieve this goal?

There are 3 factors called the 'key components of performance' that will help you achieve your desired outcomes in any area of life. These are knowledge, attitude and skill. To assist you further in achieving your outcomes and raising your awareness more around how you could be blocking yourself from creating your dreams, fill in your numbers below to see what you need to move forwards. I will give you a personal example. Score these out of 10.

My subject is online courses.

Knowledge	3
Attitude	5
Skill	4

What knowledge do I need to run an online course?

The platform to host it on.
How the content should be presented.
How to market it.
Target audience.

What skills do I need?

Research skills.
Out source what I cannot do.
Computer literacy and social media access.
Structure and process skills.

What attitude do I need to adopt to achieve my goal?

An attitude of non procrastination.
Determination.
Persistence.
Perseverance.

Why will I choose to adopt these attitudes?

Because online courses lead to a passive income which will give me more time freedom to pursue other interests in my life and allow me to spend more time with my dog and family.

Can you see how when we break a subject down into these 3 areas we start to become really aware of we need to be changing or doing so we can create our outcomes? The above leads to an in-depth list of 'how to' reach the end result. Sometimes we will need to look outside of ourselves for help and this process will allow you to recognise this process. Do you want to learn the skills needed or is it a more sensible option to out source to people who are already great at this area? People can spend a long period of time learning particular skills when it would have been quicker and more economically viable to get someone else to do it. Think about it like this, how much money do you earn per hour and if you spent 10 hours of your time learning a skill would it have been cheaper to hire someone to do it for you and spend your time generating outcomes in a different area?

Is what you are doing making economical sense?

Now have a look at your goal and see what you will need to make it happen.

What knowledge do you need?

What skills do you need?

What attitude do you need?

Why will you choose to adopt these attitudes?

Now that you have a good idea of what could have been blocking or limiting you let's put this into an action plan that is your contract with yourself to remind you daily of the choices you have now made and the actions you are going to take that will lead you to achieving your desired goal.

My Action Plan!

What qualities I will use? Who will I be? My identity.

eg: resilience, perseverance, patience. I will be strong.

What is important to me about this goal? My values.

eg: time freedom, social life, stability and security.

What I believe about myself? My beliefs.

eg: I can achieve my goal, I have strength, I have achieved in the past and can again.

My Action Plan!

What skills do I have?

eg: adaptability, discipline, computer skills, language skills, people skills.

What will I do now? My behaviours

eg: set daily time for each activity, contact people whose help I need, believe in myself.

Put this in a place where you can see it daily and remind yourself of your agreed actions that you are going to take so you will achieve your goal.

"Action is creation"

Feedback

How important is feedback?   Just think about your current day and if I asked you the question "how was your day", what would you answer?   Would you say "it was great, I achieved more than I expected, I met some lovely people, I felt good" or would you say "it was ok, it could have been better, I got stuck in traffic, I was late for a meeting, I work with miserable people"? Notice the difference between the two, how many times do you come home from work and state all the negative aspects of the day?   When people ask you how you are, do you go through a list of ailments and problems?   This is a crucial thing to recognise about ourselves because everything you say, your unconscious takes personally and makes part of your personal reality. Think about that for just a moment, if you are reciting all of the negative things that have occurred throughout the day are you feeling good or bad?   If you are focusing on everything that is not right or what went wrong, are you asking for more or less of it in the future?

If you have learnt anything so far through this book, you should have learnt that we get what we are focused on and what we are focused on grows and grows and grows.   Have you heard the old saying that you have two wolves on the inside, one wolf that is angry and negative and one wolf that is determined and positive?   The saying goes, whatever wolf you feed will grow to be big and strong, which wolf do you want to be the biggest and strongest?   There are no differences between the wolves and your thoughts, whichever you feed daily will grow to be the biggest and strongest.   Remember that the thoughts you have feed your body's chemicals which lead to your emotional states and the health of your body. What do you want to feed? How many times do you hear people respond to the question "how was your day" with a negative answer?   Out of curiosity, spend 7 days paying close attention to how people answer that question and notice what wolf they are feeding. It can be a real eye opener when you do this, you may find that you are surrounded by a majority of people who answer in the negative without be aware they are even doing so. We are all programmed and whatever programs we keep doing, our mind/body will make permanent (autopilot) so we don't have to worry about remembering to do them. Negative talk can be programmed to our autopilot system so easily because as a species we seem to have this innate need to share our pains with each other. What would happen though if we begin to interrupt each others patterns and ask specifically what went well today?

"Feedback some good"

There are some simple reasons why we look for the negative, do you remember school?   At school we are constantly tested and told what we got wrong or have our papers marked with big red X's. This takes our focus into the space of what is wrong with us or how stupid we are, not the 95% we got right and how well we did. Think of this in the context of parenting too, how many times do you hear parents telling their children "don't do that, don't touch that, stop that, don't be so stupid"? You don't know what you don't know and if we were taught to praise the positives and improve the not so goods, then we would learn a different way of being through life.

Your first task for one week is to answer the question "how are you?" with sentences that involve the opposite of a negative response. If you really have had the worst week ever how can you still reframe it to give it a different feel and change your internal perspective around it. I want you to think about sayings that are better than where you are, I am not wanting you to paint a rose garden or take yourself into the space of super duper positivity just something better. If we try to go from 0 to 100 in one go it can be too much and we can stumble before we start. Just little steps bit by bit to walk yourself out of the negative talk. This takes practice and should be considered a fun game that will raise your awareness and help your mind/body feel much better.

Examples;

"Today has been a challenge and I have made some progress"
"I am ok and working on being even better"
"The traffic was stationery so I got to listen to some good music"
"I had a lot to do and I enjoyed the challenge"
"I may have had flu, however I am emotionally good"
"I am looking to take more time out for me"

When you get the hang of softening your negatives into a better place you can them ramp them up a level. The more you do this the more you will create different patterns as auto responses to peoples enquiries about your life or situations. To be honest, tiredness is one area of my life that I use this process in, I used to say "I am knackered, tired, need sleep" and this used to lead me into the space of feeling even more tired throughout the day and sleeping 10 hours per night. Now I frame it as "I have had a full packed day and feel ready for a good recharge", the difference being now my brain is looking forward to recharging when I sleep, so I am less restless and more energised when I wake up. Some simple changes in the way we speak can lead to massive shifts in our lives.

The more you listen to yourself and pay close attention the tone of what you are saying the more you can slowly and carefully reprogram your default settings to take you into a supportive balanced space in life. We spend so much time rushing around just blurting out our programmed responses with no thought about how this is impacting us and those around us. What would happen now if you changed your current pattern, what different results would you feel at the end of the day/week?

Giving ourselves positive feedback is also a great way of motivating ourselves to do more in the future and reflecting on our journey so far. Your second task is to give yourself feedback at the end of the day and the end of the week using the following questions.

What went well?

eg: I made the calls I wanted to make, I finished 2 tasks, I felt balanced, I ate well, the kids were funny.

What can you do to take it to the next level?

eg: Meditate before work, breathe before I speak, write a list of tasks, tell myself I am doing great, spend more time focused on kids and less on my phone.

What one thing will you improve to make tomorrow even better?

eg: My attitude to tasks, the tone of my voice, my lunch choice, put my phone down.

What did I do today that I was proud of?

eg: I kept my cool, I smiled in the meeting, I changed my thoughts.

How do I feel when I have a good day?

eg: Satisfied, fulfilled, happy.

What will I do tomorrow to feel even better?

eg: Turn off snooze and enjoy the extra 20 mins sleep, smile at people on the bus, say good morning to more people, take a good lunch to work, laugh at myself more, dream about my next holiday, make someone a random cup of tea.

"Make a choice to make a difference"

Choices

For you to have a different life, you have to make different choices. So many people use the old excuse of 'I have tried that and it did not work' and the majority of these people have spent 2 days 'trying' to create a new habit and have then just given up. It has taken many years to get where you are today and you have many years left to change what is not working for you. Personal development is not a one day affair, it is a life long journey of challenges and progression. Some days you will not feel like getting out of bed at the alarm or doing the 15 minute walk instead of the drive or spending 10 minutes meditating, however, the more you do the things that will create the change when you don't feel like it, the quicker you will reach the outcomes you wish to achieve in life. Life gets easier when we do the things we procrastinate about. There is a handy tip for getting stuff done when you find yourself wandering off in the other direction, give yourself a countdown. I use this technique and you will be surprised at how successful it is in getting you to do the task you are avoiding. Imagine you are at NASA and they are giving you a countdown from 5, when you hit 1 you will jump into action, make the call, do the exercise, start the meditation, get out of bed. Try it and have some fun with it.

To become fully self supporting and happier in life takes work. It takes you making the decision to change things one by one until you are in the place of balance. It does not mean that you will never face challenges again in your life, it just means that when you do they will be easier to deal with and you will have learnt to have a different mindset towards them. Developing mental agility will allow you to overcome what in the past may have defeated you. Cultivating an internal state of finding solutions helps people to find more joy out of their daily activities, it brings with it the security and sense that you can achieve more rather than landing in the space of being a victim to life.

"Do or Do Not…. There is No Try"

And remember… if at first you don't succeed, do and do again! A result is better than no result.

References & Extras

This book contains information that I have learnt from some great teachers over the years and conclusions that I have drawn from experience. I continually challenge and contemplate my knowledge to see if it is relevant to me in the moment. We are always evolving and progressing and through this process the way we think will change. I like to revisit what I think I know to allow me to keep myself up to date and aware of how experiences challenge my perspectives. Everyday I learn something new and this process alone is proven to enhance your brain plasticity and grow new neural connections. Life is a continuous cycle of learning and when you stay in the mindset of the beginner, you will enjoy all interactions with an open mind. Those who think they know everything tend to fall the hardest and no person knows everything. It is good to master our crafts or skills, however be careful of the ego as when it appears it can limit our ability to find solutions, make choices, build relationships and progress forwards. Recognising the ego is simple it tends to rise in two main ways. Number one is the context of "what do they know?" when you hear yourself saying this on the inside just notice how you are shutting yourself off from new learning or experiences. Number two is the voice that tells you that you are "not good enough" this negative voice is also the ego. I would recommend that when you hear either kick in, you challenge them and ask yourself "how is this thought benefitting me?". Then the obvious follow up is that you get to make a choice, be directed by your ego or learn something new about yourself or someone else.

I would just like to give credit to Byron Katie, whom I have mentioned during the belief busting section of this book. This amazing lady has created a process that you can use to pull apart limiting beliefs, I would highly recommend that you google her and do the work.

The basis and foundation for what I now do in life comes from Neuro Linguistic Programming. Learning how to use your brain is a fundamental that should be taught in schools. The understanding of how your system works and the systems of other people will free you from the pattered societal chains we are all bound by. NLP was created by Richard Bandler & John Grinder and I would highly recommend researching these guys and the subject in general.

When working in the therapeutic realm I mainly use a product called 'Spectrum Emotional Coaching' this tool was developed years ago to work with removing PTSD from the system. It has a success rate of over 85% and I love using it because it is content free meaning the client does not have to talk about the past traumatic events which allows deep change to happen without revisiting trauma. It recodes emotional barcodes attached to memories which means that the person can no longer be triggered into old patterns of negative behavioural responses. Mick Stott is a remarkable man who has created an effective and efficient way of helping people move on from mild anxiety to extreme PTSD.

I work on the basis that everything has its place in the personal development realm and choosing the right tool for the right job is essential.

You wouldn't use a screwdriver to bang in a nail! However, there are some people that could bang a nail in with any tool :) There are many different processes that can be used for different purposes in relation to helping someone move forwards with life. Keep yourself open to all the options available and you may be surprised at what you find.

I wanted to share with you some of my favourite people that I love to watch on youtube or read their books. This is my personal list of some of the most impactful coaches, trainers and speakers who have inspired me to find more balance and peace which has led to me building my own businesses and finding a sense of value in my life. Enjoy!

Bruce Lipton	- Epigenetics & The Biology of Belief
Dr Joe Dispenza	- Breaking the Habit of Being Yourself
Gregg Braden	- New Human Story
Byron Katie	- The Work
Owen Fitzpatrick	- The Charismatic Edge
Bob Proctor	- The Art of Thinking
Simon Sinek	- Start With Why
Jim Rohn	- Leading an Inspired Life

Dan Pena	- Your First 100 Million
Caroline Myss	- Anatomy of the Spirit
Donna Eden	- Energy Medicine
Eckhard Tolle	- The Power of Now
Tony Robbins	- Unleash the Power Within
Mel Robbins	- The 5 Second Rule

My final thoughts are of value I always strive to give people as much value as possible from what I do. I like to make sure people are guided to the places and spaces that will benefit them and not waste valuable time or finances. For those of you wanting to know about the opportunities out there for expanding your knowledge, raising your awareness and generating successful outcomes in life and business please feel free to contact me via email or my website where I will be happy to help you decipher what it is you want that will take you to the next level. There are no shortcuts to success and loving learning will lead you continually forwards.

Making your mind matter is my mission!

"Whatever you think… you are not wrong"

Start your day in the best way. I have now created habits in my life that have changed my autopilot responses which has led to an improved inner state of peace and contentment. Following the techniques and processes in this book has helped me create more of what I want in life. Life is a continual process where there are no quick fixes. There are no magic wands or instant solutions it is a process that is never ending and takes daily practice to master. By persistently doing the little things everyday to make the difference, you can change your life. Here are my daily tips that I do to create the difference and progress towards my dreams and goals.

- wake up early
- no snooze on alarm
- heart/brain coherence meditation before starting my day
- pint of water
- 1 hours exercise
- no social media/news/tv/email/phone for first hour in the morning
- planned work activities with no distraction
- dog walk and time out
- daily reflection, planning and gratitude diary
- hot bath (reward)
- bed before 10pm

I use the heart/brain coherence meditation 3 times per day, morning, lunchtime and evening because it gives you 1800 feel good chemical hits that reduce stress, are anti ageing, anti inflammatory, immune boosting, brain enhancing and longevity generating and these last in the system for 6 hours.

Snoozing is never on the cards I much prefer to have the extra time in bed asleep rather than hitting snooze.

Drinking water first thing rehydrates the body after sleep.

Spending time exercising and creating my ideal mental state is really important rather than jumping on my phone and dealing with everyone else first. It has been proven to lower mood and productivity when you check social media or watch the news first thing in the morning. I change what I do when I exercise to keep my body on its toes and stop it getting used to the same old exercise everyday.

Planning my work sections means I get more done. I do not answer emails when I am writing programs or answer the phone when I am doing emails. Everything has its place which means I become more productive and less stressed.

I do not have an answerphone which means that no one can leave me messages I just see the missed calls and phone them back. Listening to messages can waste half hour easily and I would prefer to utilise the time for more productive activities.

Walking the dog means I get to spend time in the woods, chilling and winding down. I love the cold crisp winter days and watching the changing seasons. I switch up my routes and places so the dog and I never get bored.

Being aware of my language is high on my priority list I fully understand that every word I utter is having a direct effect on my body and creating an outcome somewhere. I focus my language on 'what I want' not 'what I don't want' this is very important because when you keep saying what you don't want you will get a shed load of it. Raising your awareness around your language can be one of the quickest ways to create massive change. Think about what you want and what you can do!

I only eat when I am hungry and stop when I no longer feel hungry, I do not eat by the clock and have been the same weight for over 20 years.

Rewarding my day with a hot bath is my favourite thing to do. I spend my bath time reflecting on the day, sending forgiveness wherever it needs to go, congratulating myself for my achievements and working out what I can do to get a better result in the future.

Doing something different every day keeps the brain in a state of plasticity. If you walk the same way to work, drive the same way, eat at the same time, drink the same drink, talk to the same people, wear the same clothes, do your hair the same way, you are just running on autopilot and will find it a massive challenge to get results in your life. I vary where I meditate, walk the dog a different route, drive different ways out of my village, change my hair, socialise in different spaces. It all helps keep me in the space of progress and helps keep me out of autopilot.

When you make small changes one by one, the compound effect of this in the future can be immense. The important thing is not to change everything all at once but just start with one simple change. To get anywhere you just have to take the first step and remember every time you fail it means you are making progress and get to improve or change what you are doing to get even better results.

I would recommend reading this book over and over because you will become more and more aware of your behaviours and autopilot responses the more you read it.

Life is not a perfect journey. I fail regularly and feel negative emotions, run old patterns and have limiting thoughts. The only difference now compared to 20 years ago is that I have knowledge, tools, techniques and awareness to help me get a different result. It wasn't easy and it is still a challenge to pursue what I want in life. I can tell you that when you make the changes and keep doing the small daily things consistently, it gets easier. Keep changing the thoughts and taking control, stop listening to others and talking rubbish to yourself. Give yourself the love that you want to feel, nurture you!

"The future is bright, the future is your choice"

Have a dream, have a goal, make it big. Limit yourself by no-one else's standards. Set your compass for a great future and keep realigning your course. No aeroplane ever fly's in a straight line but they reach their destination. Set your course and get going.

"If you want to reach your destination… set your sat-nav"

"Think big, think unlimited, dare to dream"

"Always be you because no-one else ever can be"

"Give yourself a gift of the future now"

www.wendysmith.me.uk
coachwend72@gmail.com

Made in the USA
Las Vegas, NV
20 January 2021